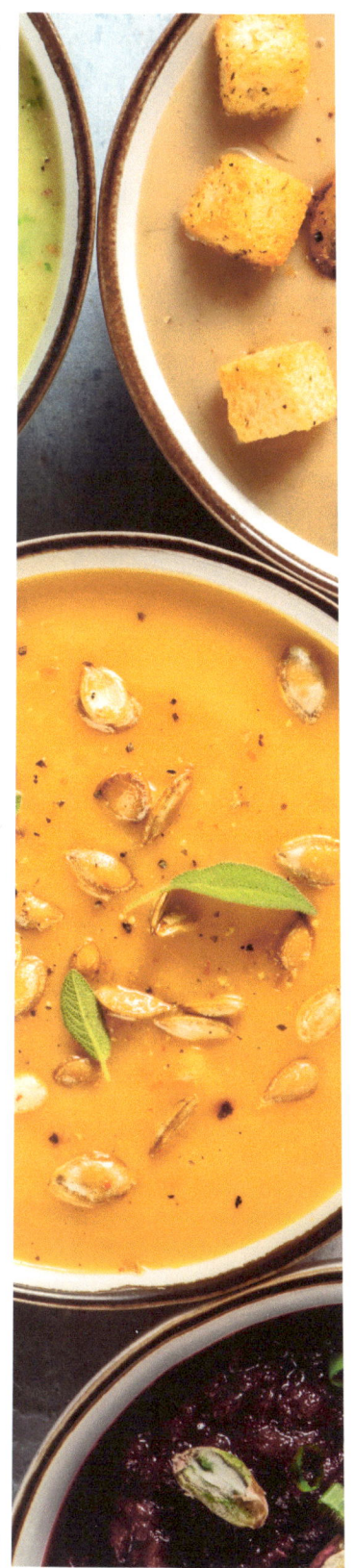

## From My Kitchen to Yours

Eating should always be a pleasure, a moment of comfort, and a means of nourishment for our bodies and souls. However, for those with no teeth or who have swallowing or chewing disorders, meal times can sometimes become a source of frustration or anxiety.

This cookbook is crafted with attention and care to bring back the joy of eating, offering delicious, nutritious, and easily consumable recipes. Whether you're looking for a hearty breakfast to start your day, a comforting lunch, a satisfying dinner, or a delightful snack, this book is designed to meet your needs, ensuring that every bite is a step towards health and happiness.

With love,
Gabrielle Harper

# BREAKFAST

*The bright start*

Breakfast is often called the most important meal of the day, and for good reason. It kickstarts your metabolism, provides your body with essential nutrients, and gives you the energy to go about your day. For those on a soft-food diet, breakfast can still be a delightful and nourishing experience.

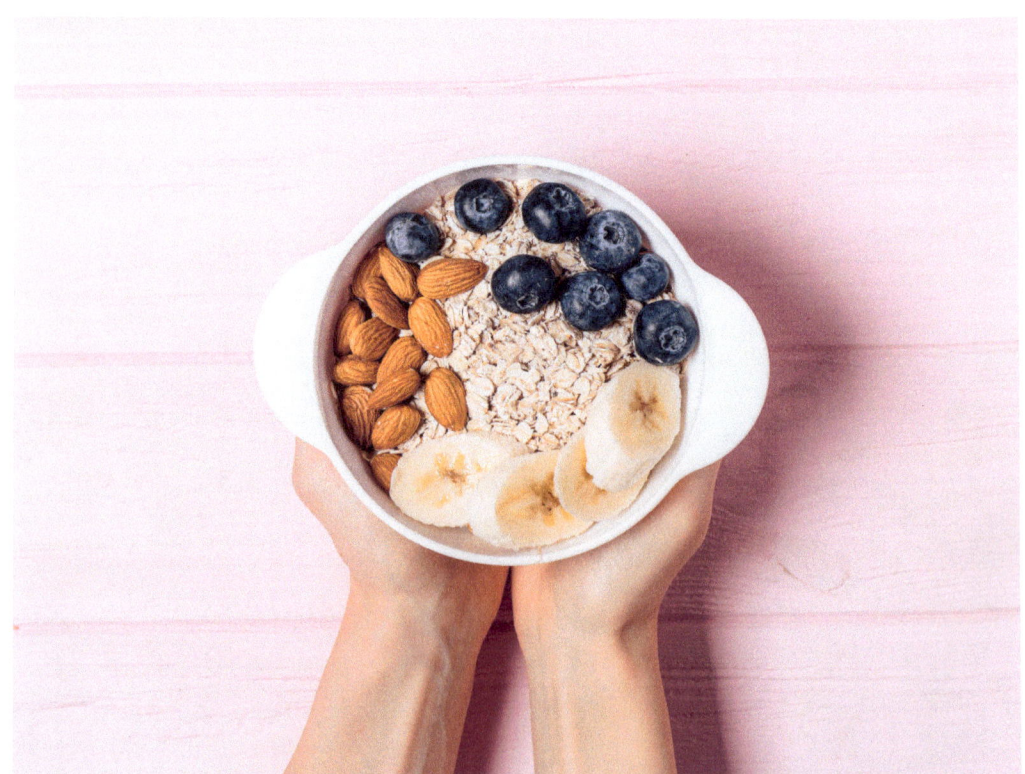

## Smoothies & Drinks

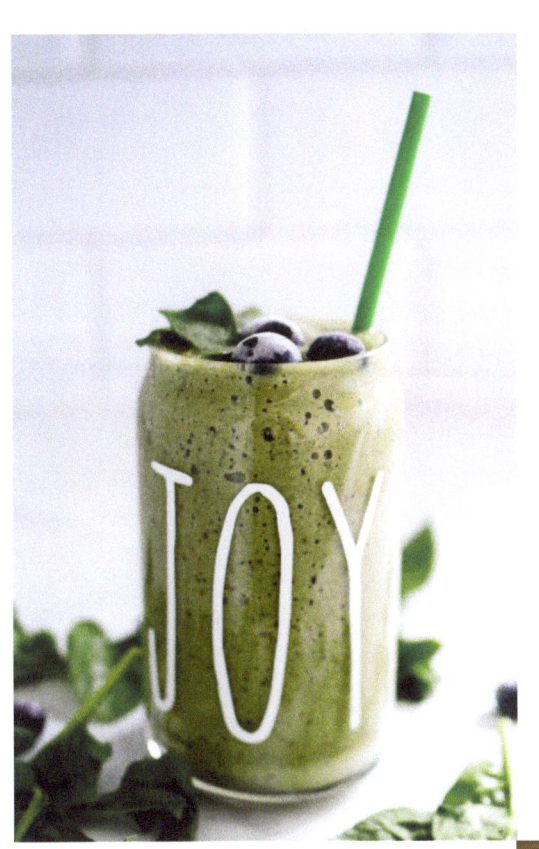

# GENTLE MORNING GREEN SMOOTHIE

### INGREDIENTS
1 cup fresh spinach leaves
1/2 ripe avocado, peeled and pitted
1 green apple, cored and sliced
1 kiwi, peeled and sliced
1 cup coconut water

Blend until smooth

# CREAMY OATMEAL BANANA SMOOTHIE

### INGREDIENTS
1/4 cup rolled oats
1 ripe banana
2 tablespoons almond butter
1 cup oat milk

Blend until smooth

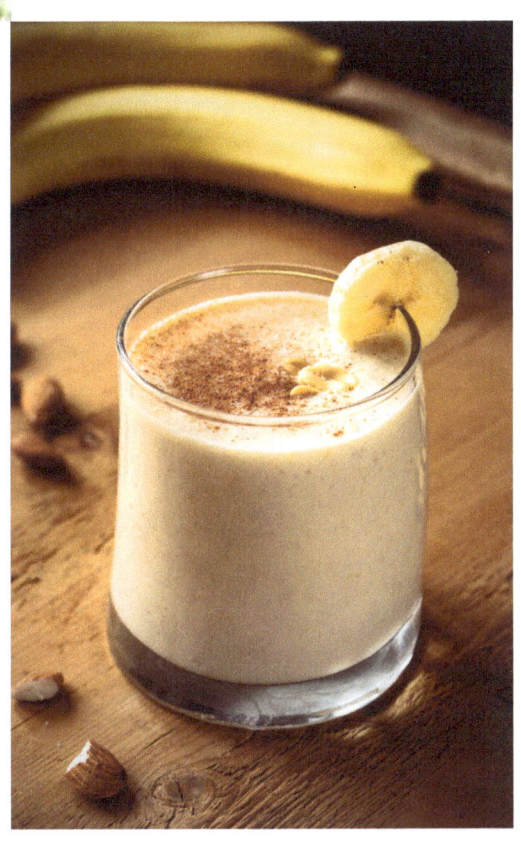

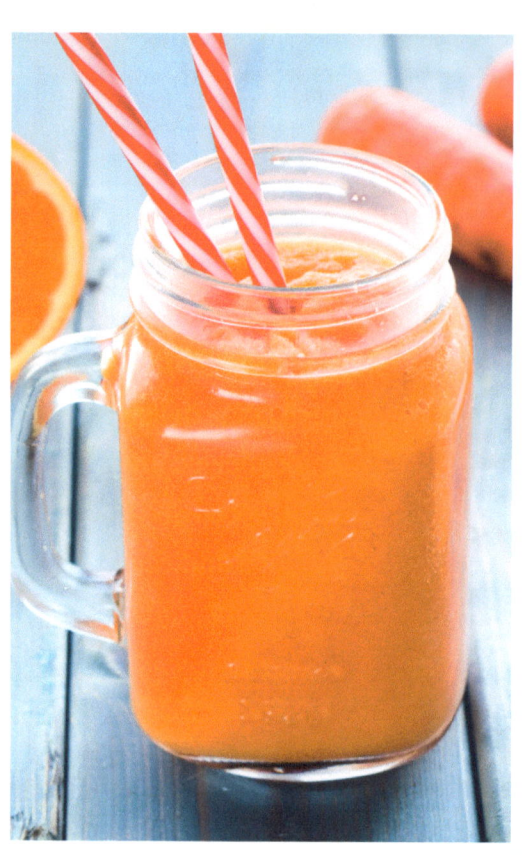

# SUNSHINE CITRUS SMOOTHIE

## INGREDIENTS

2 oranges, peeled and segmented
1 cup mango chunks, fresh or frozen
1 small carrot, peeled and chopped
1/2 teaspoon grated ginger
1 cup water or orange juice

Blend until smooth

# BLACKBERRY BLISS SMOOTHIE

## INGREDIENTS

1 cup fresh or frozen blackberries
1 medium ripe banana
1/2 cup plain Greek yogurt
1/2 cup milk
1 tablespoon honey

Blend until smooth

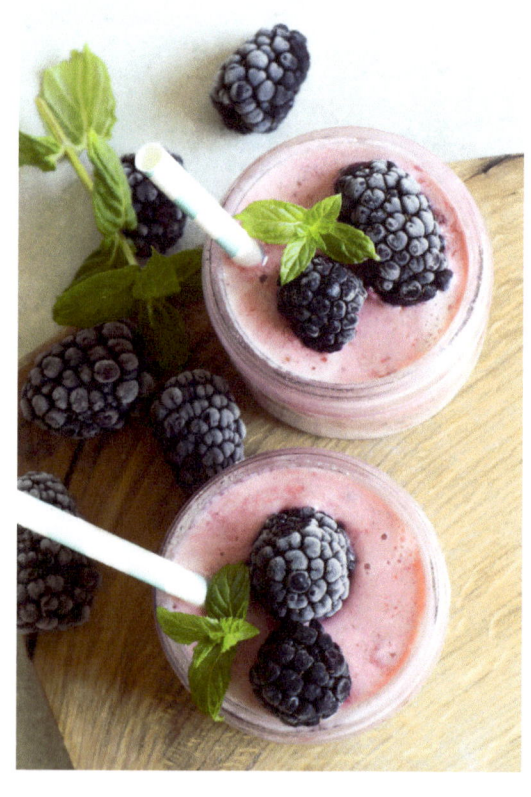

# Porridges & Cereals

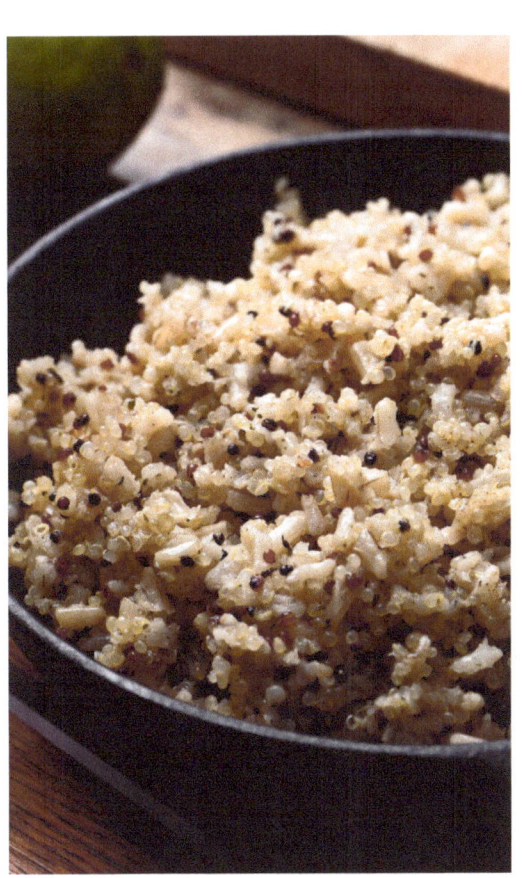

## SOOTHING QUINOA PORRIDGE

### INGREDIENTS

1/2 cup quinoa, rinsed
1 cup milk
1 apple, peeled, cored, and chopped
1/2 teaspoon cinnamon

## DIRECTIONS

1. In a small pot, combine the quinoa and milk. Bring to a boil, then reduce heat to low, cover, and simmer for 15 minutes, or until the quinoa is cooked and the liquid is mostly absorbed.
2. In another pot, stew the chopped apple with a splash of water and the cinnamon until soft and tender.
3. Serve the quinoa porridge topped with the stewed apples. Add more milk if a smoother consistency is desired.

# CREAMY COCONUT RICE PUDDING

## INGREDIENTS

1/2 cup Arborio rice
2 cups coconut milk
1 vanilla pod, split, seeds scraped
(or 1 teaspoon vanilla extract)
2 tablespoons maple syrup

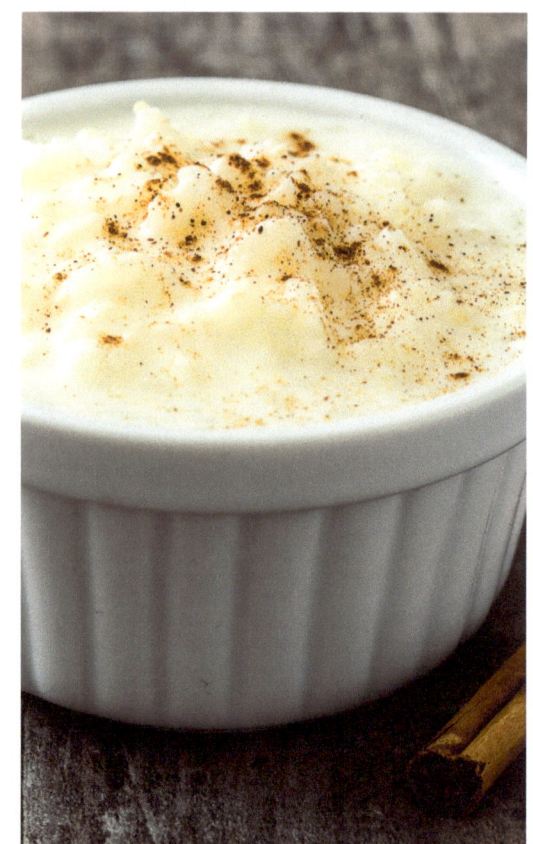

## DIRECTIONS

1. In a pot, combine the Arborio rice, coconut milk, and vanilla seeds (or extract). Bring to a gentle boil, then reduce the heat to low and simmer, stirring frequently, until the rice is tender and the mixture is creamy, about 25-30 minutes.
2. Stir in the maple syrup, adjusting the sweetness to taste.
3. Serve warm or chilled, offering a soothing and creamy dessert or breakfast option.

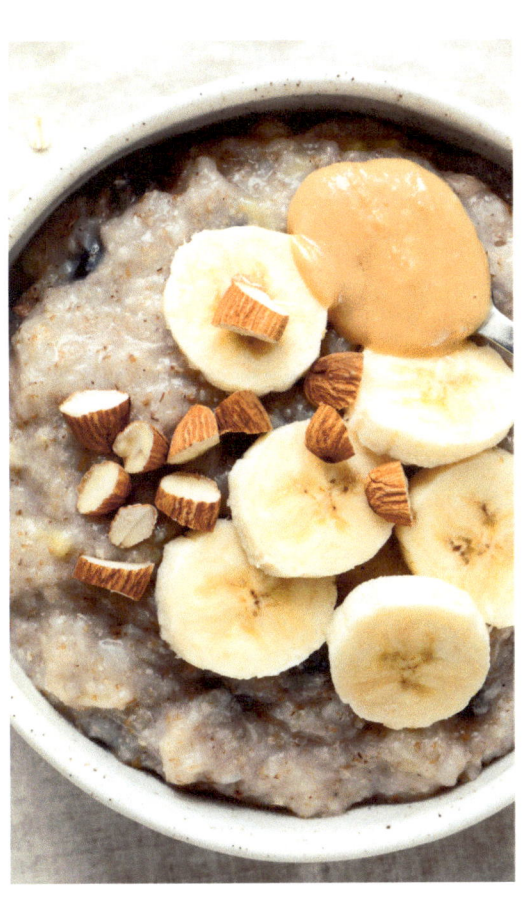

# CLASSIC WARM OATMEAL BOWL

## INGREDIENTS

1 cup rolled oats
2 cups water or milk
A pinch of salt
1/2 teaspoon cinnamon (optional)
1 tablespoon maple syrup or honey
1/2 teaspoon vanilla extract
(optional)

## DIRECTIONS

1. In a medium saucepan, bring the water or milk to a boil. Add a pinch of salt. Stir in the rolled oats and reduce the heat to medium-low. Cook, stirring occasionally, for about 5 minutes if you're using quick-cooking oats, or 10-20 minutes for old-fashioned rolled oats.
2. Stir in the maple syrup or honey, and cinnamon if desired. Taste and adjust the sweetness if necessary.
3. Pour the cooked oatmeal into a bowl. Top with your choice of fresh fruits, nuts, and seeds.

# PUMPKIN SPICE PORRIDGE

## INGREDIENTS

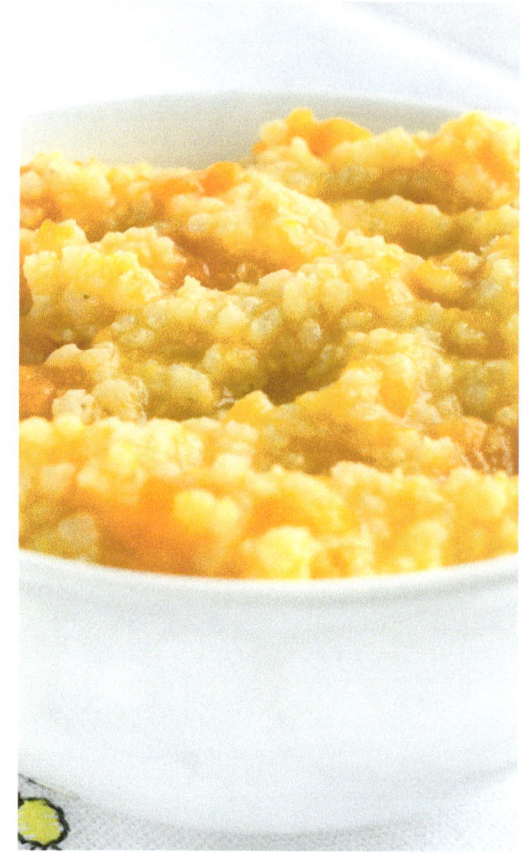

1/2 cup pumpkin puree
1 cup milk
1/4 teaspoon pumpkin pie spice
2 tablespoons maple syrup
1/2 cup instant oats

## DIRECTIONS

1. In a saucepan over medium heat, combine the pumpkin puree, milk, pumpkin pie spice, and maple syrup. Stir well.
2. Once the mixture is warm, stir in the instant oats and cook for 2-3 minutes, or until the oats are soft and the porridge is heated through.
3. Serve warm, ensuring the porridge is at a safe temperature. This porridge is a comforting, spiced breakfast that's easy to eat.

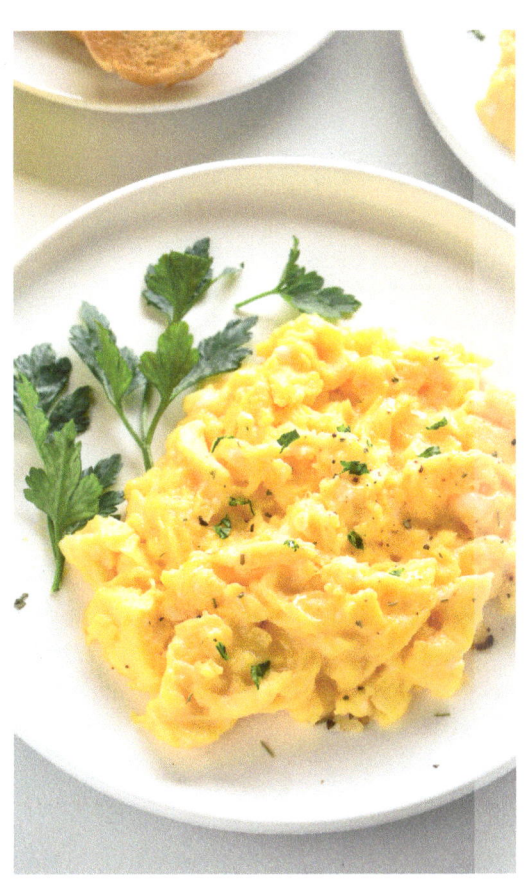

# *Egg Dishes*

## SILKY SCRAMBLED EGGS

### INGREDIENTS

3 eggs
2 tablespoons cream cheese
1 tablespoon chopped chives
A pinch of salt

## DIRECTIONS

1. Beat the eggs with the cream cheese, chives, and salt until well combined.
2. Heat a non-stick pan over low heat. Add the egg mixture, and cook gently, stirring constantly, until the eggs are softly set.
3. Serve immediately for a silky, flavorful breakfast option.

# SOFT BAKED EGG CUSTARD

## INGREDIENTS

4 eggs
2 cups milk
2 tablespoons sugar
1/2 teaspoon vanilla extract

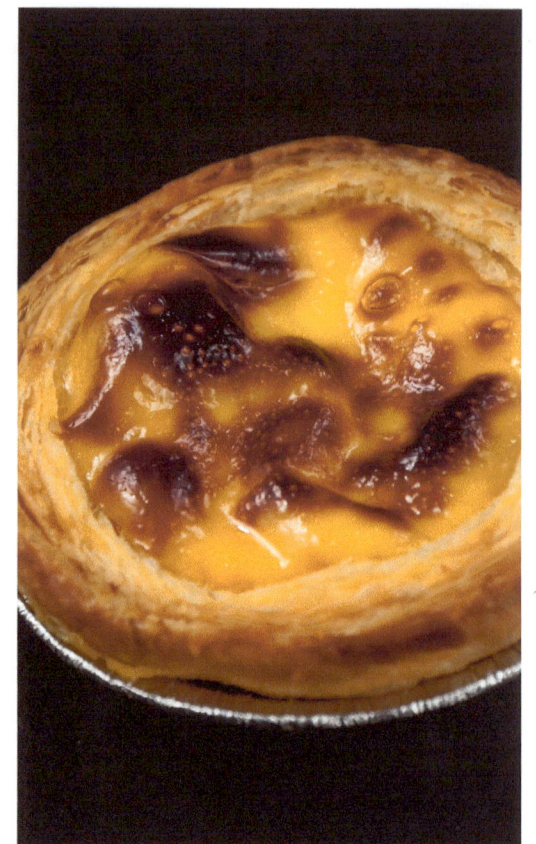

## DIRECTIONS

1. Preheat the oven to 325°F (165°C). Beat the eggs, milk, sugar, and vanilla together until well combined.
2. Pour the mixture into a baking dish. Place the dish in a larger pan and fill the pan with hot water halfway up the sides of the baking dish.
3. Bake for 45 minutes, or until the custard is just set. Allow to cool slightly before serving.

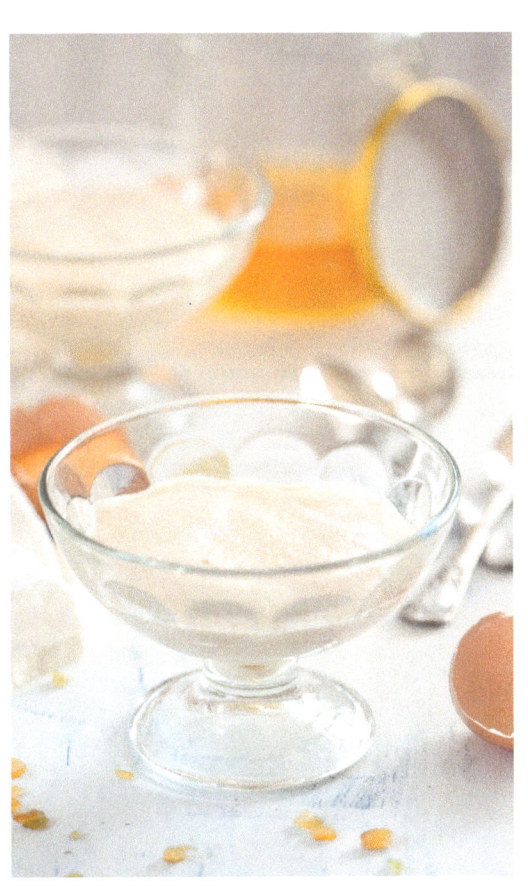

# GENTLE EGG MOUSSE

### INGREDIENTS

4 eggs, hard-boiled and peeled
1/2 cup cottage cheese
1 tablespoon chopped dill
1 teaspoon lemon zest
Salt to taste

## DIRECTIONS

1. Blend the hard-boiled eggs, cottage cheese, dill, lemon zest, and salt in a food processor until smooth.
2. Chill the mixture for at least 1 hour before serving.
3. Serve as a light spread on soft bread or crackers for an easy, nutritious snack or meal component.

# LUNCH

## *Fuel for the afternoon*

Lunch should be a time of replenishment, offering a midday boost with meals that are satisfying yet gentle for those with dietary restrictions. The recipes below focus on providing a blend of protein, vegetables, and grains that are soft and easy to consume.

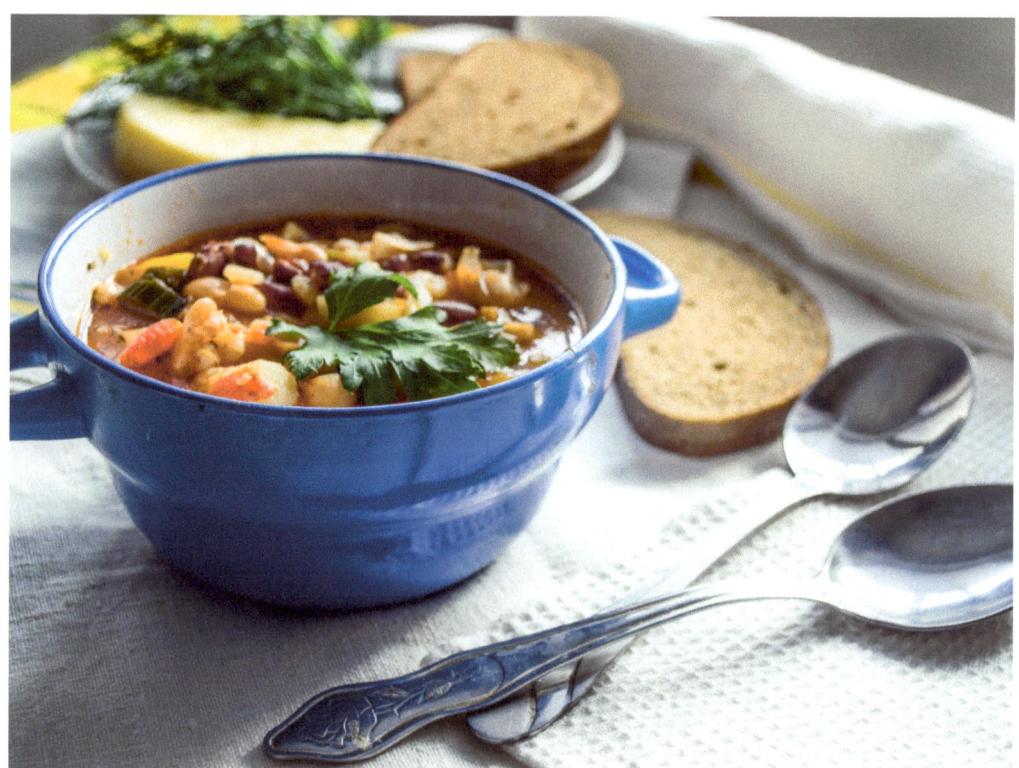

# Soups

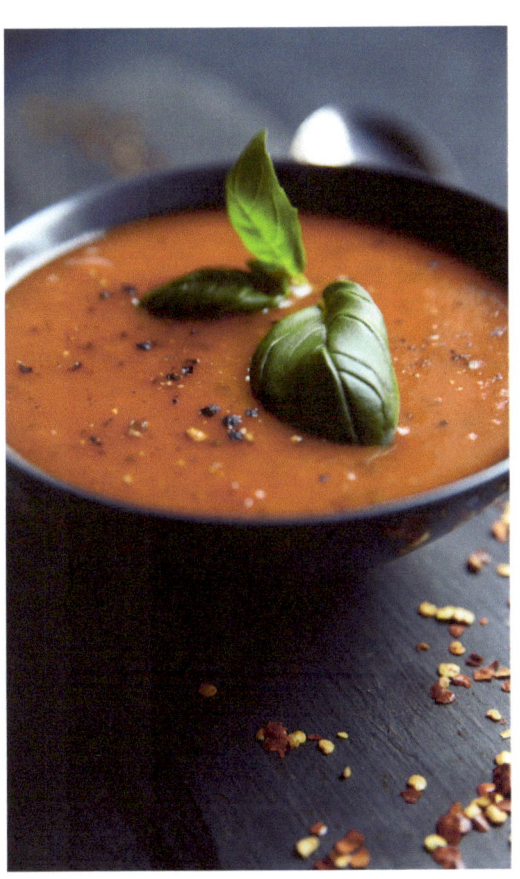

## CREAMY TOMATO BASIL SOUP

### INGREDIENTS

2 lbs ripe tomatoes, halved
4 cloves garlic, peeled
2 tablespoons olive oil
Salt and pepper, to taste
4 cups vegetable broth
1/2 cup fresh basil leaves, plus more for garnish

### DIRECTIONS

1. Preheat the oven to 400°F (200°C). Place the tomato halves and garlic cloves on a baking sheet. Drizzle with olive oil and season with salt and pepper. Roast for 25-30 minutes, until soft and slightly charred.
2. Transfer the roasted tomatoes and garlic to a large pot. Add the vegetable broth and bring to a simmer over medium heat.
3. Add the basil leaves. Using an immersion blender, puree the soup until smooth. Alternatively, you can use a regular blender, working in batches if necessary.
4. Season the soup with additional salt and pepper to taste. Serve hot, garnished with fresh basil.

# BUTTERNUT SQUASH VELVET SOUP

## INGREDIENTS

1 medium butternut squash, peeled, seeded, and chopped
2 carrots, peeled and chopped
1 tablespoon olive oil
4 cups vegetable broth
1 cup coconut milk
1/2 teaspoon ground cinnamon
Salt and pepper, to taste

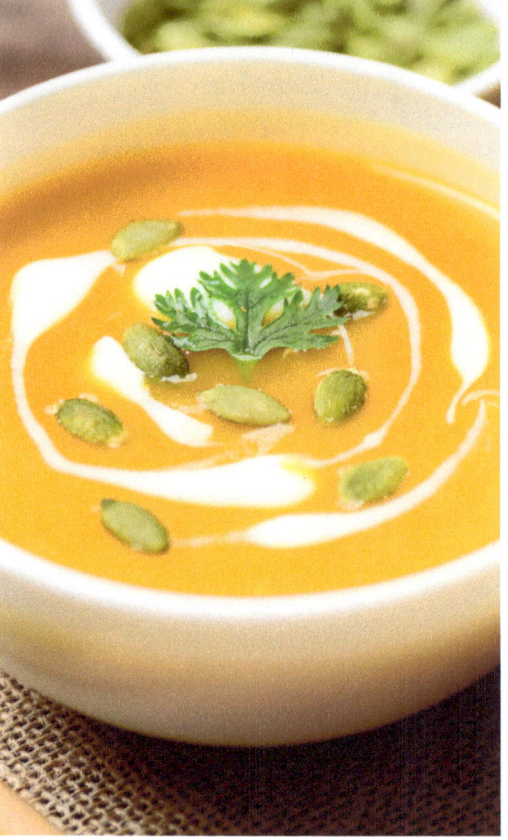

## DIRECTIONS

1. In a large pot, heat the olive oil over medium heat. Add the chopped butternut squash and carrots. Cook, stirring occasionally, for about 10 minutes or until slightly softened.
2. Add the vegetable broth and bring the mixture to a boil. Reduce heat and simmer for about 20 minutes or until the vegetables are very soft.
3. Stir in the coconut milk and ground cinnamon. Using an immersion blender, puree the soup until completely smooth.
4. Season with salt and pepper to taste. Serve warm, offering a creamy, comforting bowl of soup.

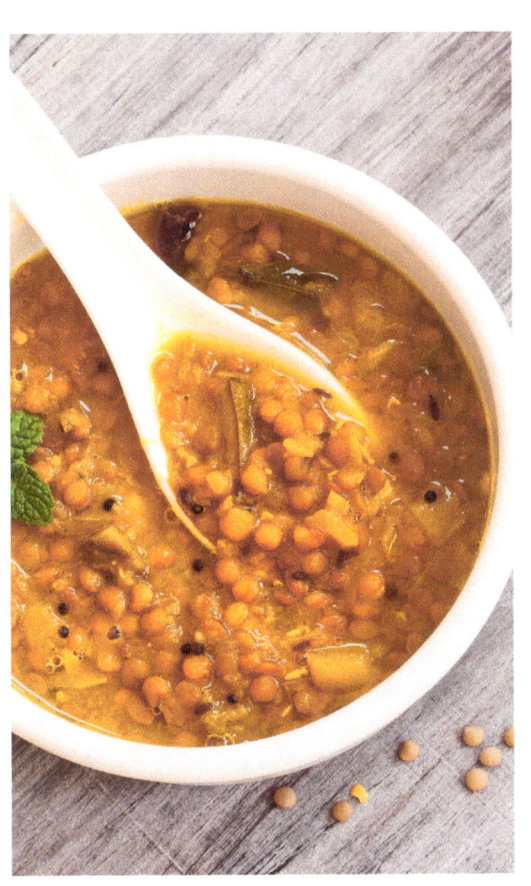

# SOFT LENTIL SOUP

## INGREDIENTS

1 cup red lentils, rinsed
2 carrots, peeled and chopped
2 stalks celery, chopped
1 onion, chopped
2 cloves garlic, minced
1 tablespoon olive oil
4 cups vegetable broth
1 teaspoon dried thyme
Salt and pepper, to taste

## DIRECTIONS

1. In a large pot, heat the olive oil over medium heat. Add the onion, carrots, celery, and garlic. Sauté until the vegetables are softened, about 5 minutes.
2. Add the rinsed lentils and vegetable broth to the pot. Stir in the dried thyme.
3. Bring the mixture to a boil, then reduce the heat and simmer for about 20 minutes, or until the lentils are soft and cooked through.
4. Using an immersion blender, puree the soup until smooth. Season with salt and pepper to taste.
5. Serve hot, ensuring a smooth and comforting meal that's easy on the palate.

# Purees & Mashes

## SILKEN CAULIFLOWER MASH

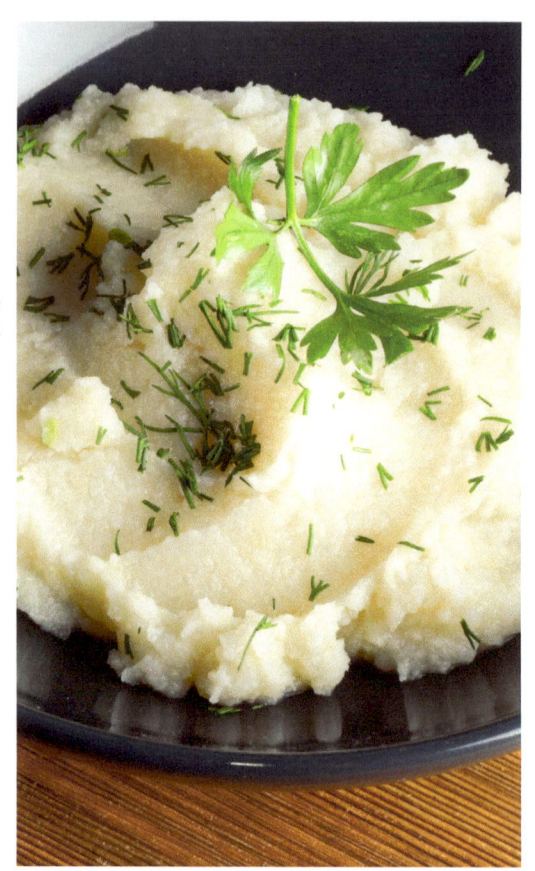

### INGREDIENTS

1 large head cauliflower, cut into florets
2 cloves garlic, minced
2 tablespoons olive oil, garlic-infused for extra flavor
1/4 cup grated Parmesan cheese
Salt and pepper, to taste

## DIRECTIONS

1. Steam the cauliflower florets until very tender, about 15 minutes.
2. In a blender or food processor, combine the steamed cauliflower, minced garlic, olive oil, and grated Parmesan cheese. Blend until smooth and creamy.
3. Season with salt and pepper to taste. Serve warm, as a delicious and nutritious alternative to traditional mashed potatoes.

# SWEET POTATO AND CARROT PUREE

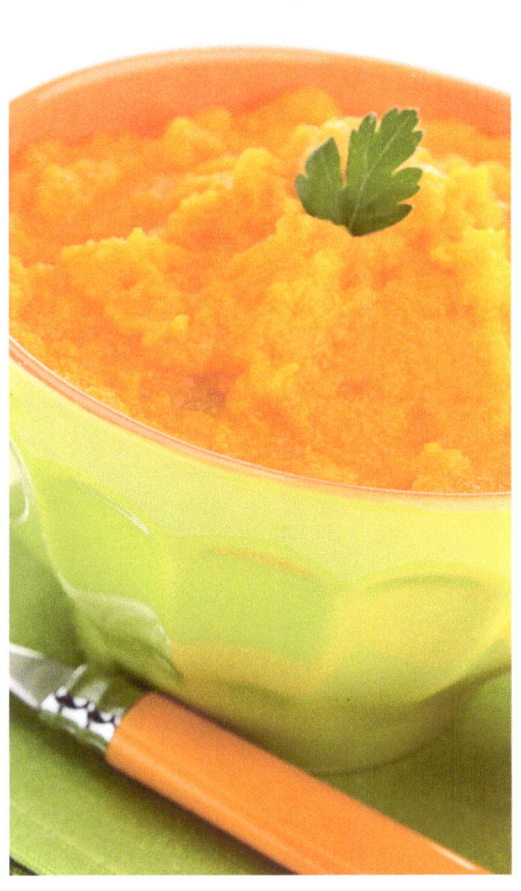

### INGREDIENTS

2 large sweet potatoes, peeled and chopped
3 carrots, peeled and chopped
1 tablespoon olive oil
1/2 teaspoon grated ginger
1 tablespoon maple syrup
Salt and pepper, to taste

## DIRECTIONS

1. Preheat the oven to 400°F (200°C). Toss the sweet potatoes and carrots with olive oil and spread them on a baking sheet. Roast for 25-30 minutes or until very tender.
2. Transfer the roasted vegetables to a blender. Add the grated ginger and maple syrup. Blend until smooth.
3. Season with salt and pepper to taste. Serve warm, offering a sweet and savory side dish rich in flavor and nutrients.

# CREAMY AVOCADO AND PEA MASH

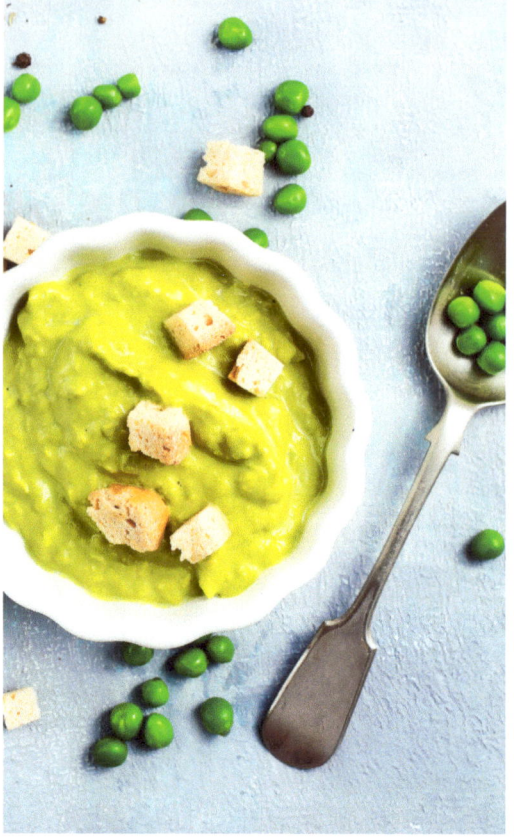

## INGREDIENTS

1 ripe avocado
1 cup green peas, cooked and cooled
1 tablespoon fresh mint leaves, chopped
Juice of 1/2 lemon
Salt and pepper, to taste

## DIRECTIONS

1. In a bowl, mash the avocado using a fork. Add the cooked green peas and continue to mash until you reach a creamy, yet slightly chunky consistency.
2. Stir in the chopped mint leaves and lemon juice. Season with salt and pepper to taste.
3. Serve as a refreshing side dish or a spread on soft, whole-grain toast.

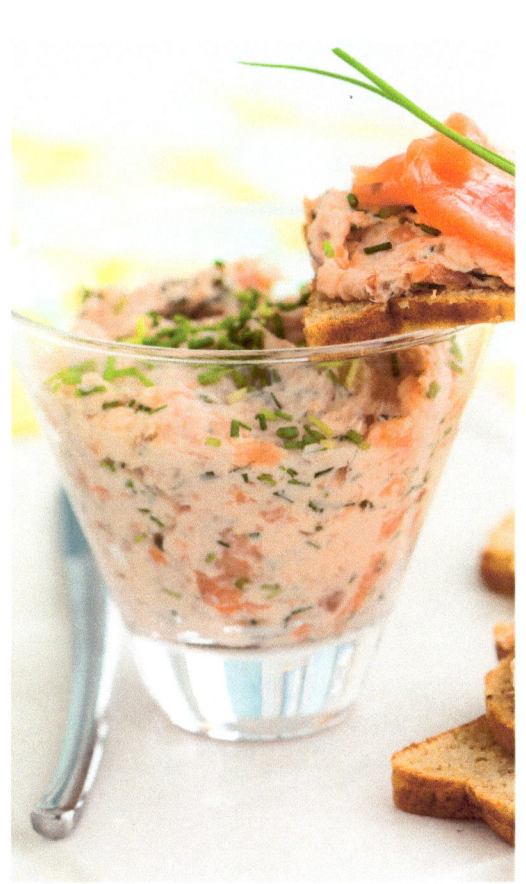

# Protein Dishes

## TENDER SALMON MOUSSE

### INGREDIENTS

8 oz cooked salmon, skin and bones removed
1/4 cup cream cheese, softened
1 tablespoon fresh dill, chopped
2 teaspoons lemon juice
Salt and pepper, to taste

## DIRECTIONS

1. In a food processor, combine the cooked salmon, cream cheese, dill, and lemon juice. Blend until smooth.
2. Season with salt and pepper to taste. Chill in the refrigerator for at least 1 hour before serving.
3. Serve as a soft spread on crackers or cucumber slices, offering a protein-rich, flavorful dish.

# CHICKEN AND VEGETABLE PUREE

## INGREDIENTS

1 boneless, skinless chicken breast, cooked and chopped
1/2 cup cooked carrots
1/2 cup cooked peas
1/2 cup chicken broth, more if needed
Salt and pepper, to taste

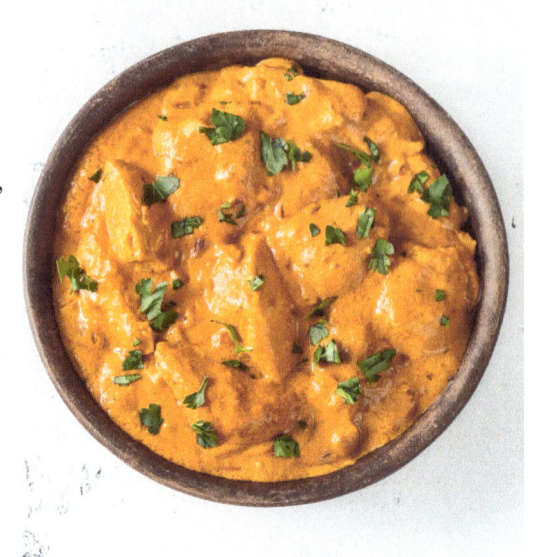

## DIRECTIONS

1. In a blender or food processor, combine the cooked chicken, carrots, peas, and chicken broth. Blend until smooth, adding more broth as needed to reach the desired consistency.
2. Season with salt and pepper to taste. Serve warm, ensuring a nutritious and easily consumable meal.

# SOFT BEEF AND MUSHROOM RAGOUT

## INGREDIENTS

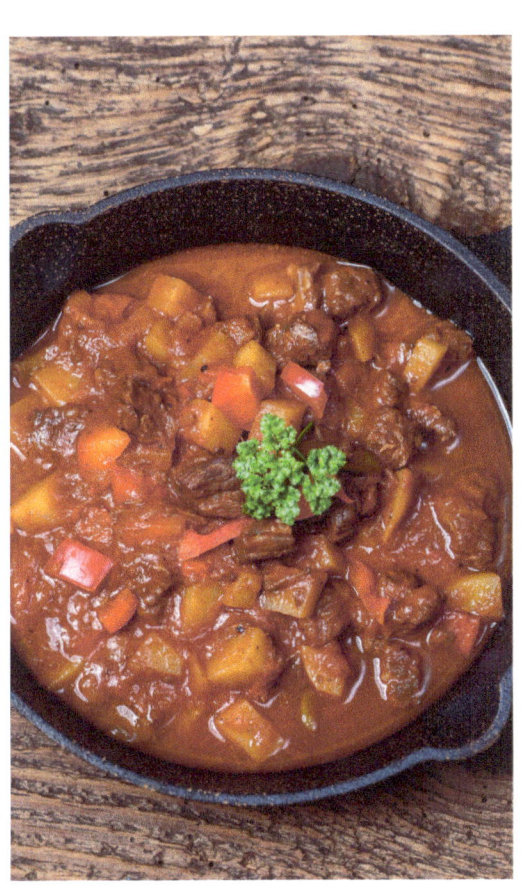

1 lb beef stew meat, cooked until very tender
1 cup mushrooms, cooked
1 onion, cooked until soft
2 cups beef broth
Salt and pepper, to taste
1 tablespoon fresh parsley, chopped (optional)

## DIRECTIONS

1. In a large pot, add the beef stew meat and cover it with water. Bring to a boil, then reduce the heat to a simmer. Allow the beef to cook until it is very tender
2. In a skillet over medium heat, add the chopped onions and mushrooms and cook until soft. Stir occasionally to prevent sticking.
3. In a blender or food processor, combine the cooked beef, softened mushrooms, and onions. Add 1 cup of beef broth and blend until smooth.

# NOURISHING EGG SALAD

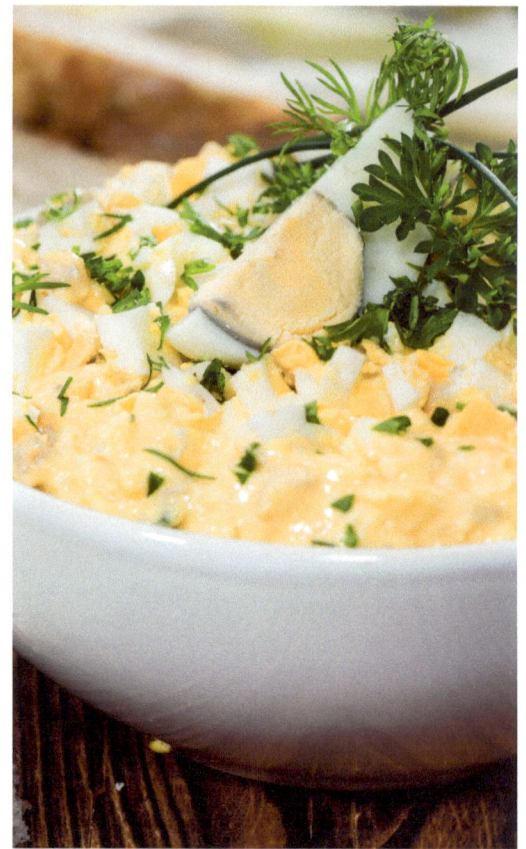

## INGREDIENTS

6 hard-boiled eggs, peeled
1/4 cup mayonnaise
2 tablespoons mustard
Salt and pepper, to taste
Paprika (optional)

## DIRECTIONS

1. In a bowl, mash the hard-boiled eggs with a fork or potato masher until smooth.
2. Stir in the mayonnaise and mustard until well combined. Season with salt and pepper to taste.
3. Serve chilled, garnished with a sprinkle of paprika for added color and flavor if desired.
4. Can be served on its own or with soft bread if tolerated.

# CHICKEN AND RICE PORRIDGE

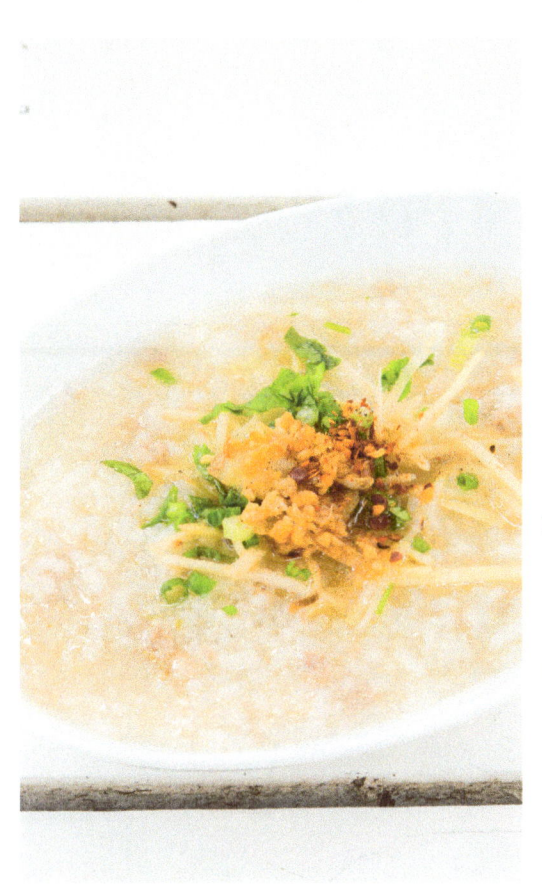

## INGREDIENTS

1/2 cup rice, rinsed
1 boneless, skinless chicken breast
6 cups water or chicken broth
Salt, to taste
Optional garnishes: green onions, ginger (finely minced), soy sauce

## DIRECTIONS

1. Combine the rice, chicken breast, and water or broth in a large pot. Bring to a boil, then reduce heat to a simmer.
2. Cook until the chicken is fully cooked and the rice has broken down into a porridge consistency, about 1-1.5 hours. Stir occasionally to prevent sticking.
3. Remove the chicken, shred it finely or blend it, then return it to the pot. Season with salt to taste.
4. Serve hot, garnished with optional green onions and ginger, with soy sauce on the side for added flavor. Ensure the porridge is smooth and easy to eat.

# DINNER

## *The comfort gathering*

Dinner is a time for relaxation and nourishment. These recipes provide the body with essential nutrients to repair and rejuvenate overnight, featuring soft, easy-to-digest ingredients that are perfect for a soothing end to the day.

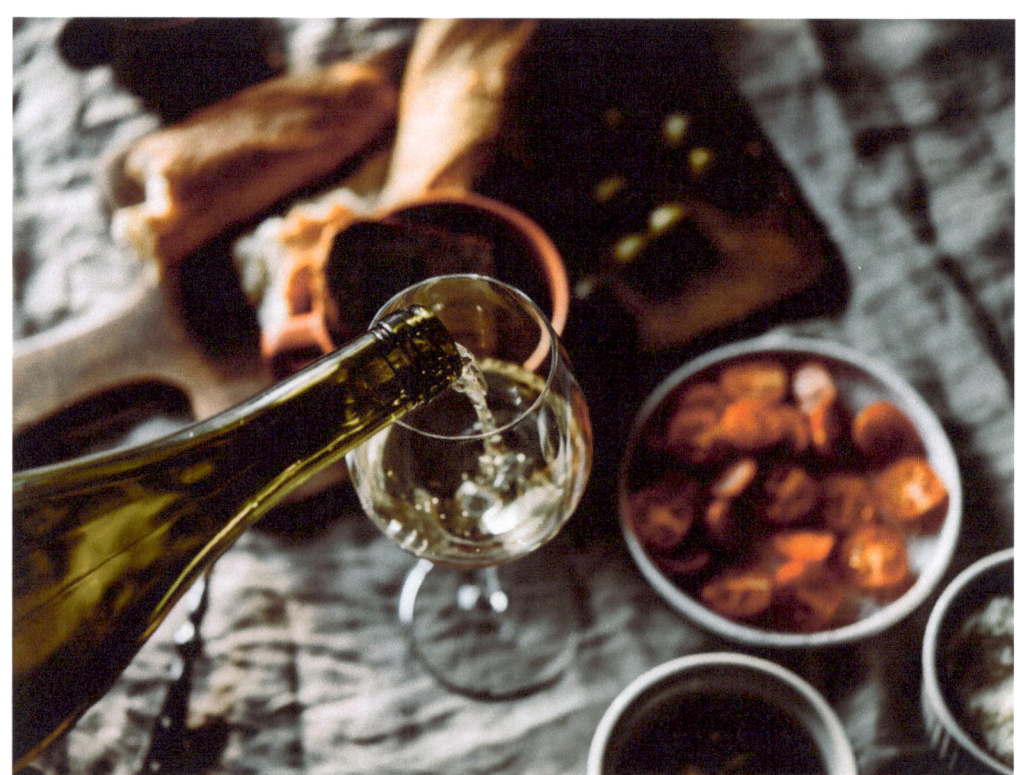

# Stews & Casseroles

## CHICKEN AND VEGETABLE STEW

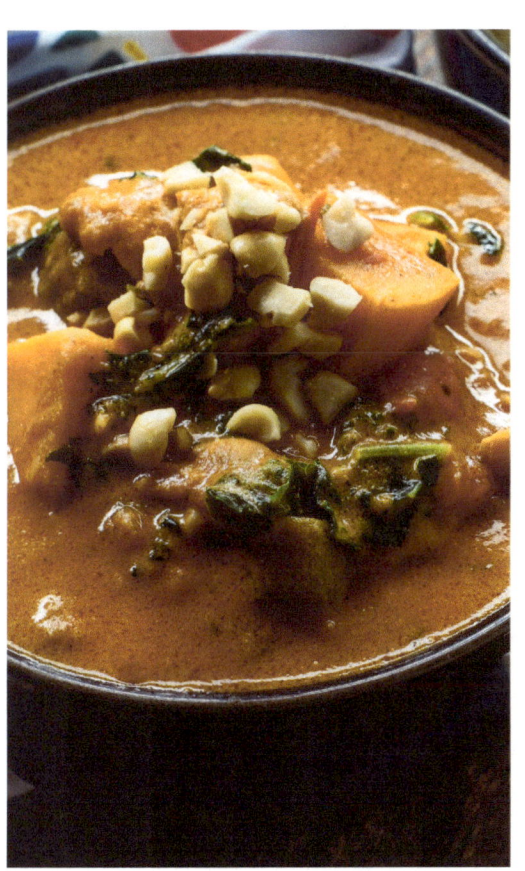

### INGREDIENTS

2 lbs chicken thighs, boneless and skinless
2 carrots, peeled and chopped
2 zucchinis, chopped
2 potatoes, peeled and chopped
4 cups chicken broth
1 cup heavy cream
Salt and pepper, to taste
2 tablespoons olive oil

## DIRECTIONS

1. In a large pot, heat the olive oil over medium heat. Add the chicken thighs and cook until browned on all sides.
2. Add the chopped carrots, zucchinis, and potatoes to the pot. Pour in the chicken broth and bring to a simmer.
3. Cover and simmer on low heat for about 1 hour, or until the vegetables are very soft and the chicken is fully cooked.
4. Stir in the heavy cream and simmer for an additional 10 minutes. Season with salt and pepper.
5. Use an immersion blender to puree the stew directly in the pot until it reaches a creamy consistency. Adjust seasoning if necessary.

# LENTIL AND VEGETABLE CASSEROLE

## INGREDIENTS

1 cup green lentils, rinsed
2 cups mixed vegetables (carrots, bell peppers, zucchini), chopped
1 can (14 oz) crushed tomatoes
2 garlic cloves, minced
1 onion, chopped
2 teaspoons dried Italian herbs
Salt and pepper, to taste
2 tablespoons olive oil
2 cups vegetable broth

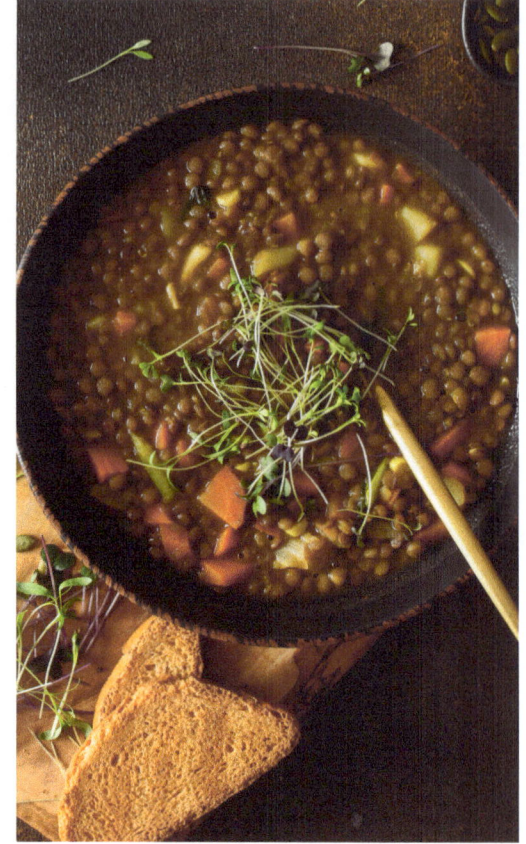

## DIRECTIONS

1. Preheat your oven to 375°F (190°C). In a skillet, heat the olive oil over medium heat. Add the onion and garlic, cooking until soft and fragrant.
2. Stir in the crushed tomatoes, mixed vegetables, rinsed lentils, Italian herbs, and vegetable broth. Bring to a simmer, then season with salt and pepper.
3. Transfer the mixture to a casserole dish. Cover with aluminum foil and bake for about 45 minutes, or until the lentils are fully cooked and soft.
4. After baking, blend the casserole using an immersion blender until it reaches a smooth consistency.

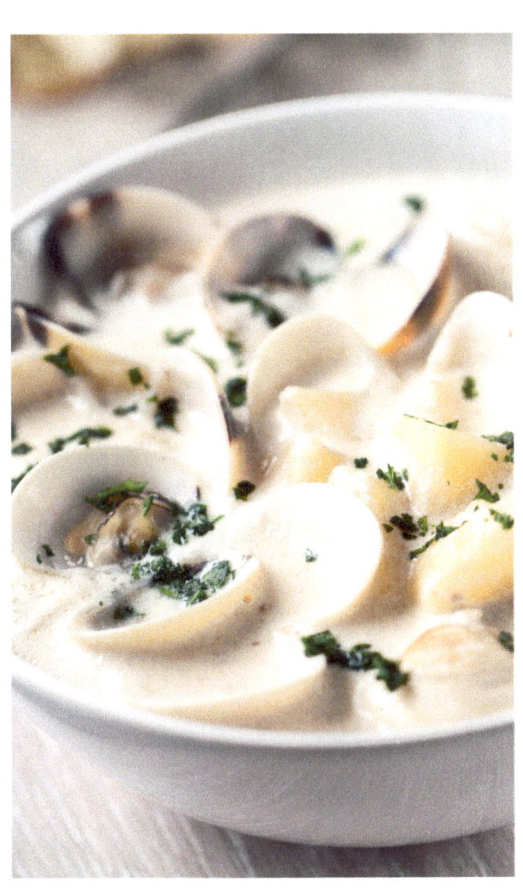

# SOOTHING SEAFOOD CHOWDER

## INGREDIENTS

1 lb mixed seafood (shrimp, scallops, and any firm white fish), chopped
2 potatoes, peeled and diced
1 cup corn kernels, fresh or frozen
1 onion, chopped
2 cups fish or vegetable broth
1 cup heavy cream
Salt and white pepper, to taste
2 tablespoons butter

## DIRECTIONS

1. In a large pot, melt the butter over medium heat. Add the chopped onion and cook until translucent.
2. Add the diced potatoes and broth. Bring to a boil, then reduce heat and simmer until the potatoes are tender.
3. Stir in the seafood and corn. Cook until the seafood is just cooked through, about 5-7 minutes.
4. Reduce the heat to low and stir in the heavy cream. Season with salt and white pepper.
5. Use an immersion blender to carefully blend the chowder until it is smooth.

# Soft Veggies

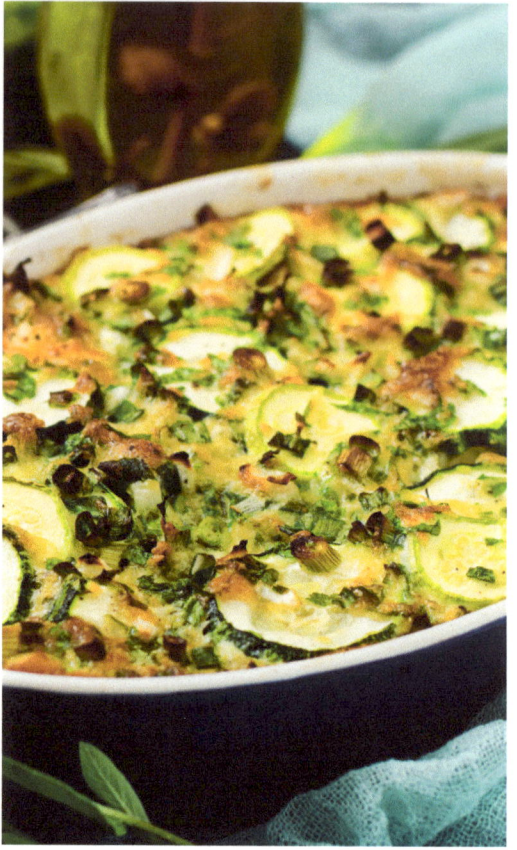

## ZUCCHINI AND SQUASH RIBBON CASSEROLE

### INGREDIENTS

2 zucchinis
2 yellow squashes
1 cup ricotta cheese
Salt and pepper, to taste
1/2 cup grated Parmesan cheese

## DIRECTIONS

1. Preheat your oven to 350°F (175°C). Using a vegetable peeler or mandoline, slice the zucchinis and yellow squashes into thin ribbons.
2. In a mixing bowl, combine the ricotta cheese with salt and pepper.
3. Layer the zucchini and squash ribbons in a baking dish, alternating with spoonfuls of the ricotta mixture.
4. Sprinkle the top with grated Parmesan cheese. Cover with foil and bake for 20-25 minutes, or until the vegetables are very soft.
5. Blend the casserole lightly with an immersion blender to achieve a soft, easily consumable consistency.

# CARROT AND PARSNIP PUREE

## INGREDIENTS

4 carrots, peeled and chopped
4 parsnips, peeled and chopped
1/4 cup heavy cream
1/4 teaspoon ground nutmeg
Salt and pepper, to taste
2 tablespoons butter

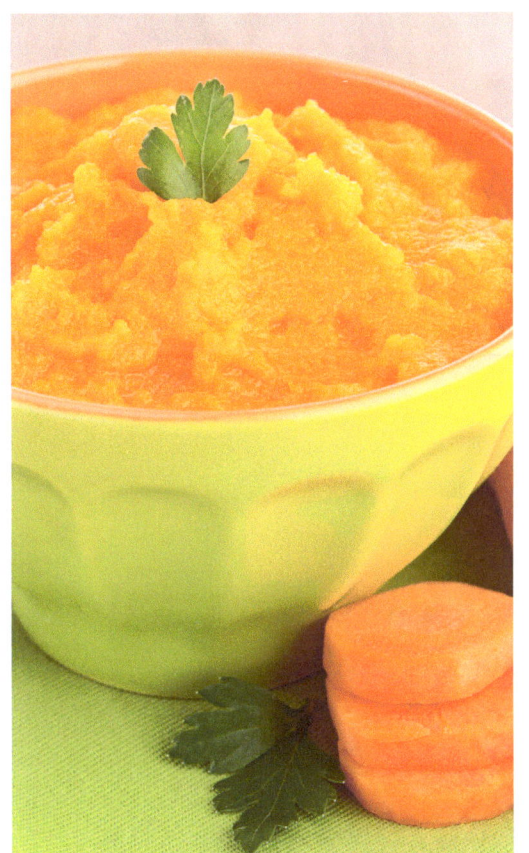

## DIRECTIONS

1. Steam the carrots and parsnips until very soft, about 15-20 minutes.
2. Transfer the steamed vegetables to a blender. Add the heavy cream, butter, nutmeg, salt, and pepper.
3. Blend until smooth and creamy. Adjust seasoning if necessary.
4. Serve warm as a sweet and savory side dish, ensuring a smooth texture that's easy to eat.

# BROCCOLI AND CAULIFLOWER CHEESE BAKE

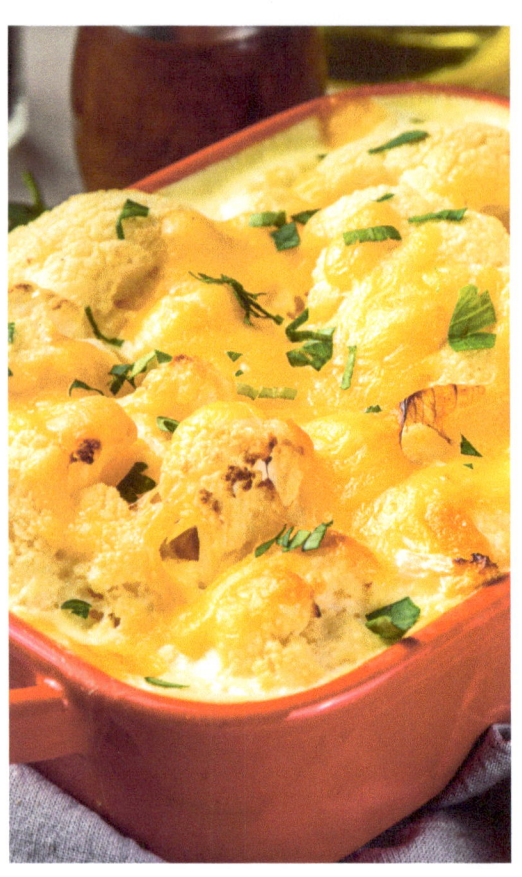

## INGREDIENTS

1 head broccoli, cut into florets
1 head cauliflower, cut into florets
2 cups cheddar cheese, shredded
1 cup milk
2 tablespoons flour
2 tablespoons butter
Salt and pepper, to taste

## DIRECTIONS

1. Steam the broccoli and cauliflower florets until very tender, about 15-20 minutes.
2. In a saucepan, melt the butter and stir in the flour to make a roux. Gradually whisk in the milk until the mixture is smooth and thickened.
3. Add 1 1/2 cups of the cheddar cheese to the sauce, stirring until melted. Season with salt and pepper.
4. Combine the steamed vegetables and cheese sauce in a baking dish. Sprinkle the remaining cheddar cheese on top.
5. Bake at 350°F (175°C) for 20-25 minutes, until the cheese is bubbly and golden.
6. Blend the bake lightly with an immersion blender to achieve a soft, creamy consistency.

# Gentle Grains

## POLENTA WITH MUSHROOM RAGOUT

### INGREDIENTS

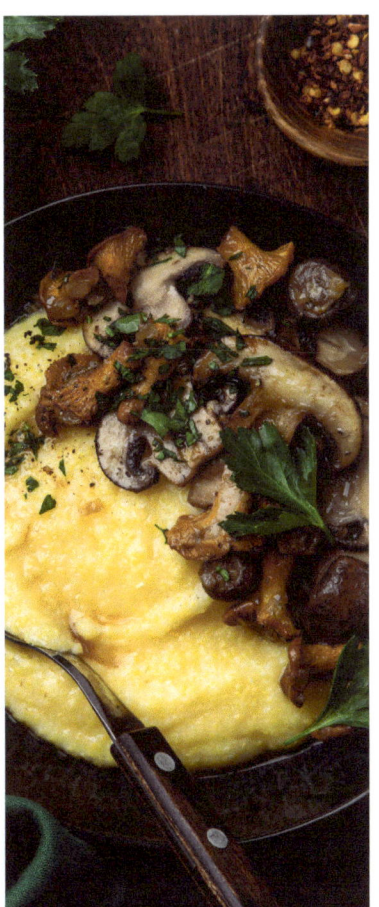

*For Polenta*
- 1 cup polenta (cornmeal)
- 4 cups water or chicken broth
- 1/2 cup grated Parmesan cheese
- 2 tablespoons butter
- Salt, to taste

*For Mushroom Ragout*
- 2 cups mushrooms, sliced (any variety)
- 2 cloves garlic, minced
- 1 onion, finely chopped
- 1 teaspoon fresh thyme, chopped
- 1 cup vegetable broth
- 2 tablespoons olive oil
- Salt and pepper, to taste

### DIRECTIONS

1. **For the Polenta:** In a large saucepan, bring the water or chicken broth to a boil. Gradually whisk in the polenta, stirring constantly to prevent lumps.
2. Reduce the heat to low and cook, stirring frequently, until the polenta is thickened and tender, about 20-30 minutes. Stir in the butter and grated Parmesan cheese until well combined. Season with salt to taste.
3. **For the Mushroom Ragout:** While the polenta is cooking, heat the olive oil in a skillet. Add the onion and garlic, sautéing until soft.
4. Add the sliced mushrooms and thyme, cooking until the mushrooms are browned. Pour in the broth, bringing the mixture to a simmer. Cook until the liquid is slightly reduced, about 10 minutes. Season with salt and pepper.
5. Use an immersion blender to lightly blend the mushroom ragout into a smoother consistency, being careful to retain some texture.

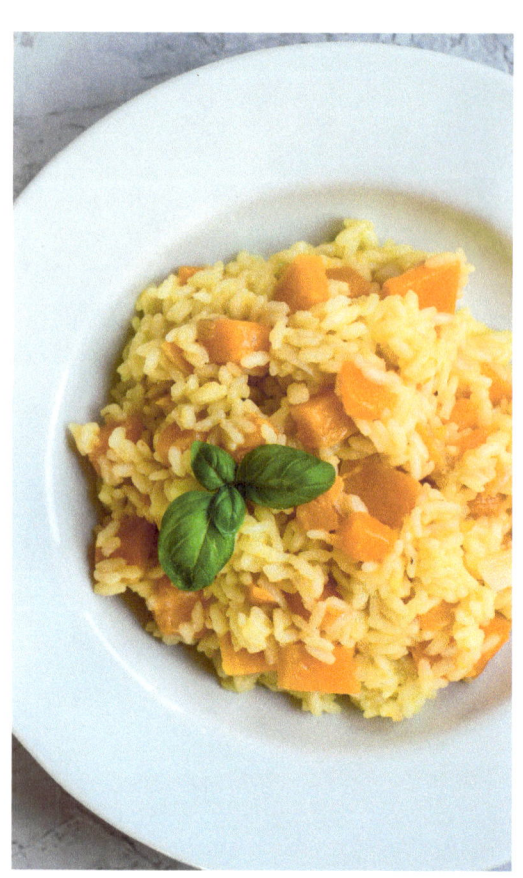

# BAKED RISOTTO WITH PUMPKIN

## INGREDIENTS

1 cup Arborio rice
2 cups pumpkin puree (canned or homemade)
4 cups vegetable broth, warmed
1 onion, finely chopped
1/2 cup grated Parmesan cheese
2 tablespoons olive oil
Salt and pepper, to taste

## DIRECTIONS

1. Preheat the oven to 375°F (190°C).
2. In a skillet, heat the olive oil. Add the onion and cook until translucent.
3. Add the Arborio rice, stirring to coat the grains with oil. Cook for 1-2 minutes.
4. Stir in the pumpkin puree and warmed vegetable broth. Season with salt and pepper.
5. Transfer the mixture to a baking dish. Cover with foil and bake in the preheated oven for 25-30 minutes, or until the liquid is absorbed and the rice is tender.
6. Stir in the grated Parmesan cheese until melted and mixed thoroughly.
7. Before serving, blend slightly with an immersion blender to ensure the risotto is soft enough to eat easily, but still has some texture.

# QUINOA AND VEGETABLE STUFFED PEPPERS

## INGREDIENTS

4 bell peppers
1 cup quinoa, cooked
1 cup spinach, chopped and sautéed
1/2 cup shredded mozzarella cheese
1/2 cup tomato sauce
1/2 cup vegetable broth
1 onion, finely chopped
2 cloves garlic, minced
2 tablespoons olive oil
Salt and pepper, to taste

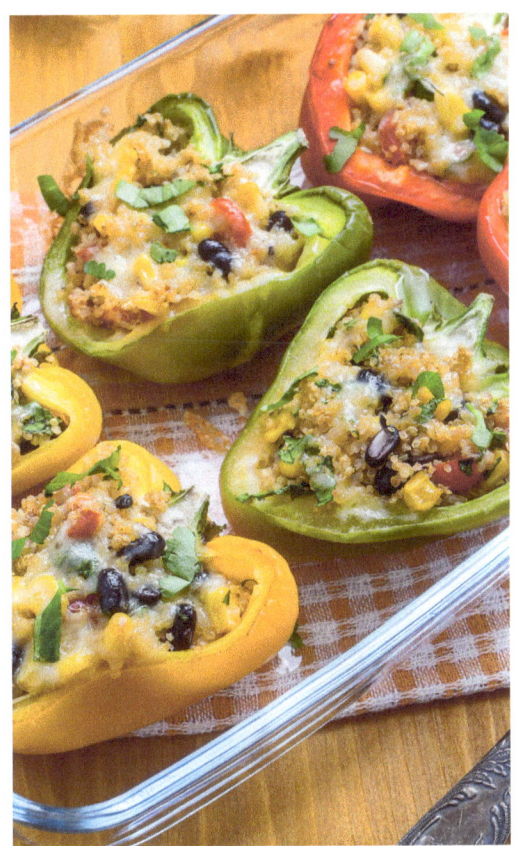

## DIRECTIONS

1. Preheat the oven to 350°F (175°C).
2. In a skillet, cook the onion and garlic with olive oil until soft.
3. In a large bowl, combine the cooked quinoa, sautéed spinach, half of the mozzarella cheese, and the onion-garlic mixture. Season with salt and pepper to taste.
4. Stuff the prepared bell peppers with the quinoa mixture. Place the stuffed peppers in a baking dish.
5. Pour the tomato sauce and vegetable broth into the bottom of the dish around the peppers. This will help keep them moist while baking.
6. Cover with foil and bake for about 30-35 minutes, or until the peppers are tender.
7. Sprinkle the remaining mozzarella cheese over the peppers and bake uncovered for an additional 5 minutes.
8. Before serving, lightly puree the contents of each pepper to ensure they are soft enough for easy consumption.

# SNACKS & DESSERTS

## *Happy little moments*

Snacks and desserts offer a moment of indulgence and satisfaction. These recipes focus on providing that pleasure through textures and flavors that are easily enjoyed, ensuring each treat is both delightful and digestible.

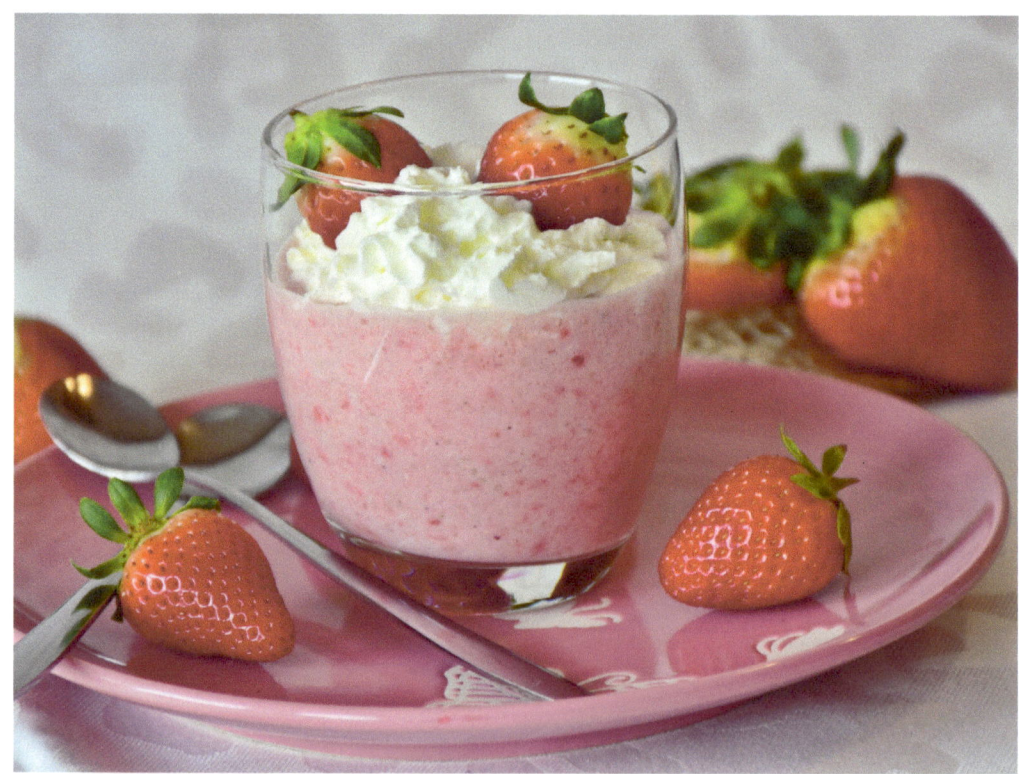

*Puddings & Mousses*

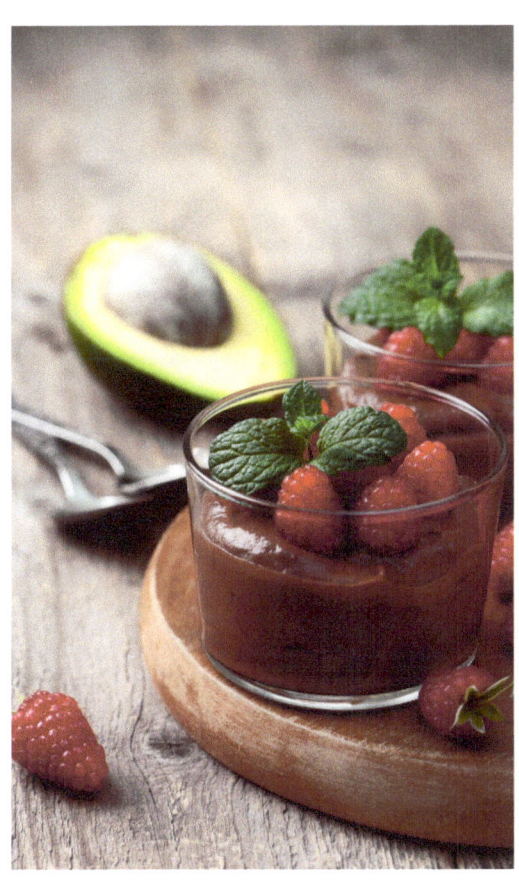

## AVOCADO CHOCOLATE MOUSSE

### INGREDIENTS

2 ripe avocados, peeled and pitted
1/4 cup cocoa powder
1/4 cup honey or maple syrup
(adjust to taste)
1 teaspoon vanilla extract
A pinch of salt
Optional: Whipped cream and berries for garnish

## DIRECTIONS

1. In a blender or food processor, combine the avocados, cocoa powder, honey (or maple syrup), vanilla extract, and a pinch of salt.
2. Blend until the mixture is smooth and creamy. Taste and adjust sweetness if needed.
3. Divide the mousse into serving dishes and refrigerate for at least 1 hour to set.
4. Serve chilled, garnished with whipped cream and berries if desired.

# VANILLA AND HONEY RICE PUDDING

## INGREDIENTS

1/2 cup Arborio rice
4 cups whole milk
1/4 cup honey
1 vanilla bean, split and seeds scraped (or 1 teaspoon vanilla extract)
A pinch of salt

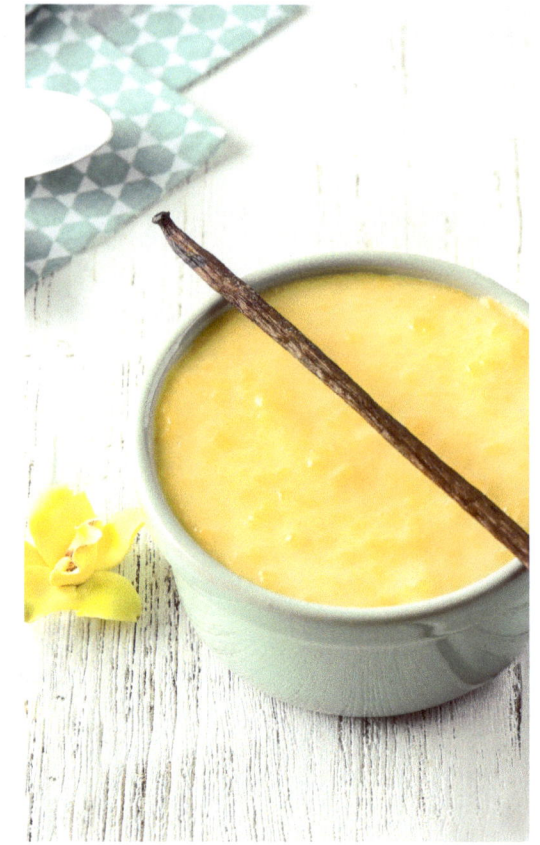

## DIRECTIONS

1. In a saucepan, combine the milk, Arborio rice, honey, vanilla bean seeds (and pod if using), and a pinch of salt.
2. Bring to a simmer over medium heat, then reduce heat to low. Cook, stirring frequently, until the rice is tender and the mixture has thickened, about 30-35 minutes.
3. Remove the vanilla bean pod (if used) and let the pudding cool slightly. It will continue to thicken as it cools.
4. Serve warm or chilled, according to preference.

# BERRY AND CHIA SEED PUDDING

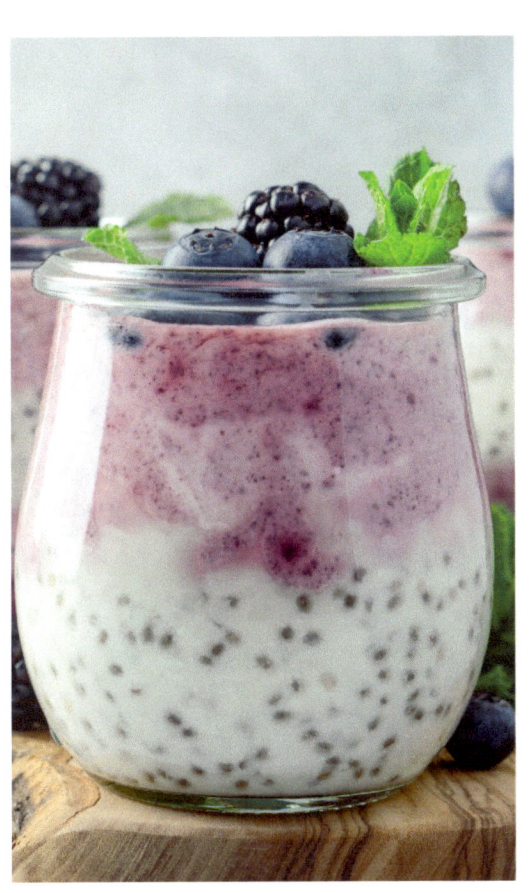

## INGREDIENTS

1/4 cup chia seeds
1 cup milk
1 cup mixed berries, mashed (reserve some for topping)
2 tablespoons honey or maple syrup
1/2 teaspoon vanilla extract

## DIRECTIONS

1. In a bowl, mix together the chia seeds, milk, mashed berries, honey (or maple syrup), and vanilla extract. You can use a blender if you prefer.
2. Stir well to combine, then cover and refrigerate for at least 4 hours, preferably overnight, until the pudding has thickened.
3. Stir the pudding before serving. Add more milk if it's too thick. Top with the reserved berries.

# *Baked Goods*

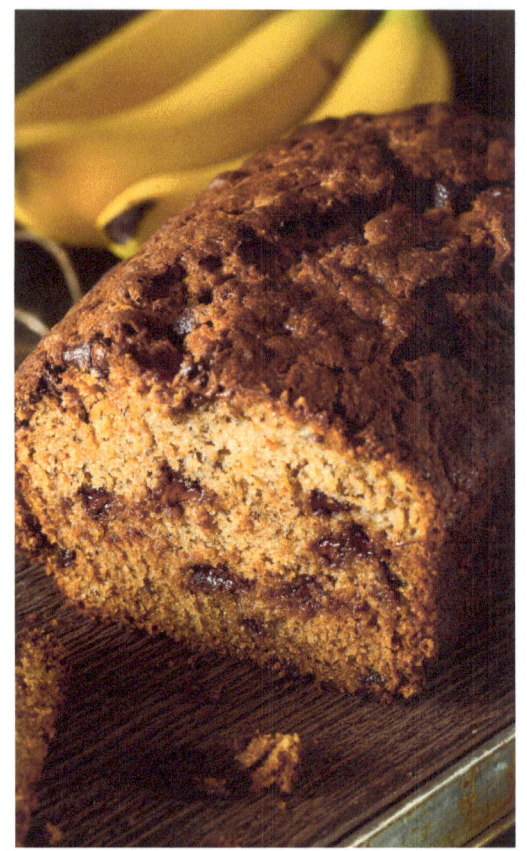

## MOIST BANANA BREAD

### INGREDIENTS

3 very ripe bananas, mashed
1/3 cup melted butter
1/2 cup sugar
1 egg, beaten
1 teaspoon vanilla extract
1 teaspoon baking soda
A pinch of salt
1 1/2 cups all-purpose flour

## DIRECTIONS

1. Preheat your oven to 350°F (175°C). Grease a 4x8-inch loaf pan.
2. In a mixing bowl, combine the mashed bananas with melted butter. Stir in the sugar, beaten egg, and vanilla extract.
3. Sprinkle the baking soda and salt over the mixture, then add the flour. Stir until just combined.
4. Pour the batter into the prepared loaf pan. Bake for 50-60 minutes, or until a tester inserted into the center comes out clean.
5. Let the bread cool, then blend slightly to achieve a softer consistency if desired before serving.

# APPLE SAUCE MUFFINS

## INGREDIENTS

1 cup apple sauce
1/4 cup vegetable oil
1/2 cup sugar
1 egg
1 teaspoon vanilla extract
1 teaspoon cinnamon
1 teaspoon baking soda
A pinch of salt
1 1/2 cups whole wheat flour

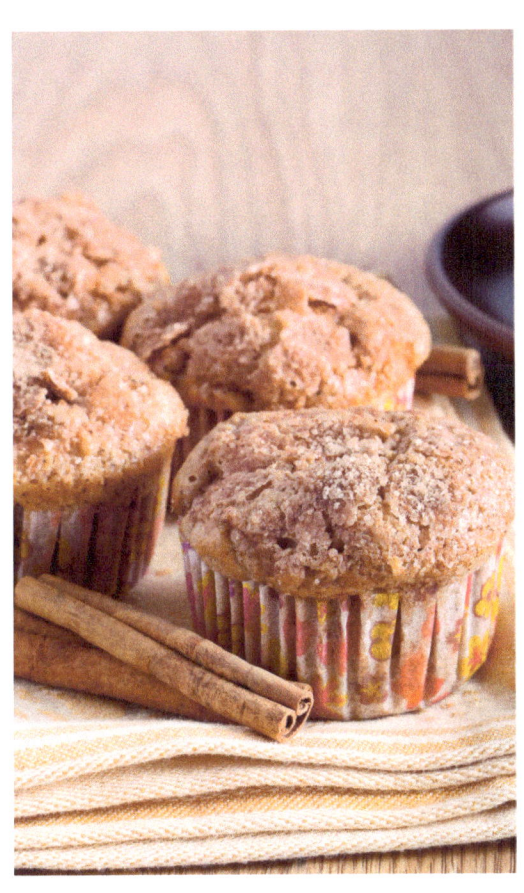

## DIRECTIONS

1. Preheat the oven to 350°F (175°C). Line a muffin tin with paper liners.
2. In a bowl, mix the apple sauce, oil, sugar, egg, and vanilla extract.
3. Add the cinnamon, baking soda, and salt. Mix well.
4. Gradually add the flour, stirring until just combined.
5. Fill the muffin tins and bake for 18-20 minutes, or until a toothpick comes out clean.
6. Once cooled, blend the muffins slightly to soften further if needed for easier consumption.

# PUMPKIN SPICE SOFT COOKIES

## INGREDIENTS

1 cup pumpkin puree
1/2 cup sugar
1/4 cup vegetable oil
1 egg
1 tablespoon pumpkin pie spice
1 teaspoon vanilla extract
1 teaspoon baking powder
1 teaspoon baking soda
A pinch of salt
2 cups all-purpose flour

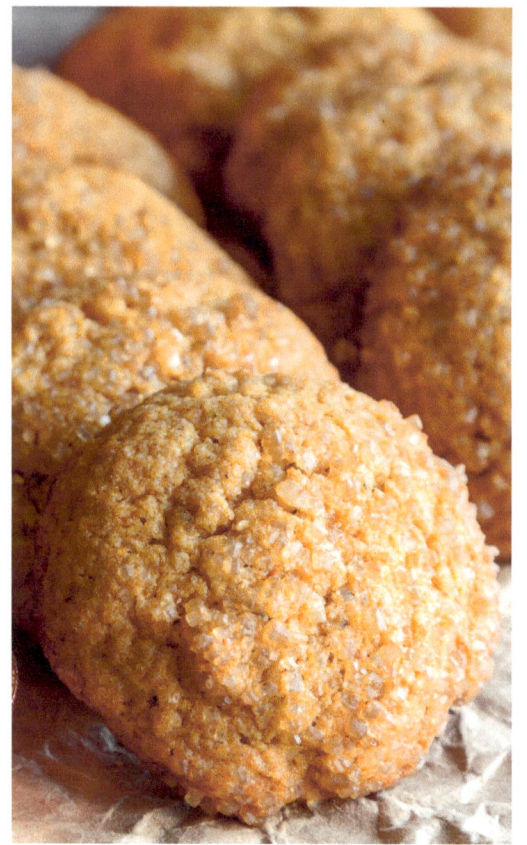

## DIRECTIONS

1. Preheat the oven to 350°F (175°C) and line a baking sheet with parchment paper.
2. In a large bowl, mix together the pumpkin puree, sugar, oil, and egg. Stir in the pumpkin pie spice, vanilla, baking powder, baking soda, and salt.
3. Gradually add the flour, mixing until just combined.
4. Drop spoonfuls of the dough onto the prepared baking sheet. Bake for 10-12 minutes or until the cookies are set.
5. Allow the cookies to cool, then lightly mash or blend for a softer texture.

*Creamy Dips & Spreads*

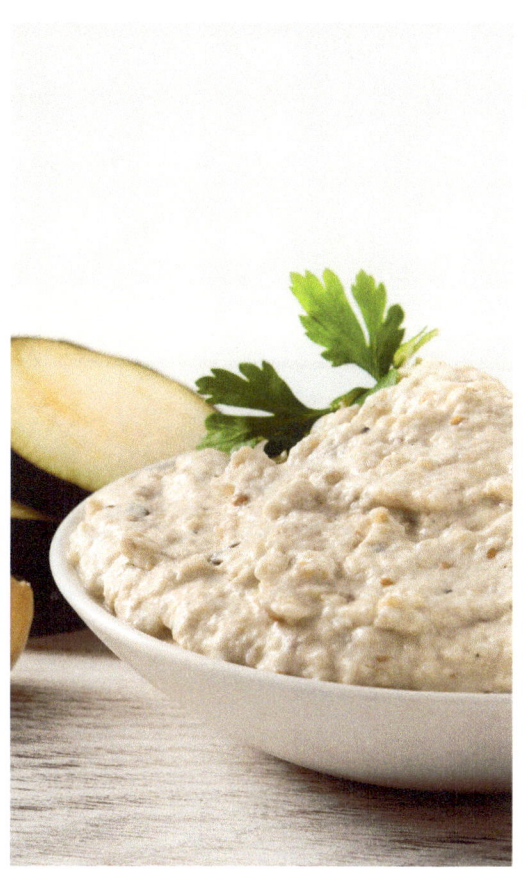

## ROASTED EGGPLANT SPREAD

### INGREDIENTS

1 large eggplant
2 cloves garlic
2 tablespoons tahini
2 tablespoons olive oil
Juice of 1 lemon
Salt and pepper, to taste

## DIRECTIONS

1. Preheat the oven to 400°F (200°C). Prick the eggplant with a fork and place it on a baking sheet along with the garlic cloves. Roast until the eggplant is very soft, about 30-40 minutes.
2. Let the eggplant cool, then peel and add the flesh to a blender along with the roasted garlic, tahini, olive oil, and lemon juice. Blend until smooth.
3. Season with salt and pepper. Serve the spread with soft, fresh bread or as a dip for vegetables.

# PEA AND MINT DIP

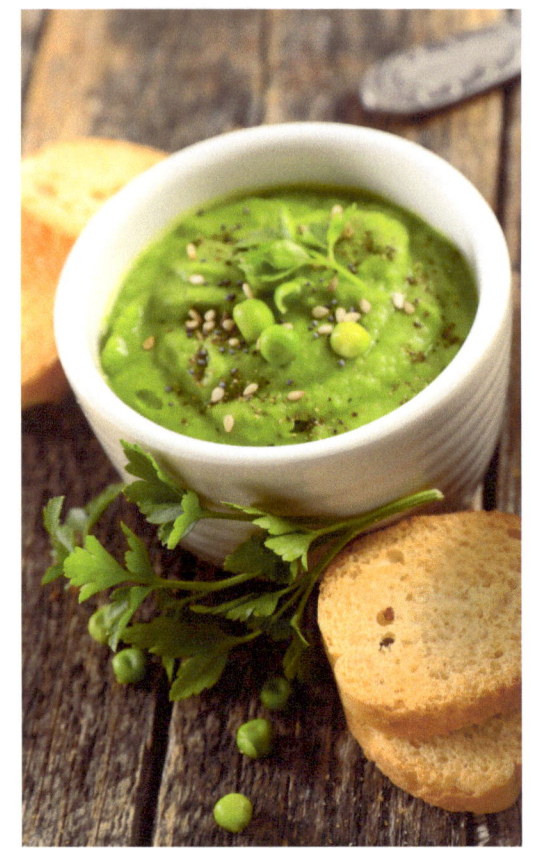

## INGREDIENTS

2 cups frozen peas, thawed
1/4 cup fresh mint leaves
1/2 cup Greek yogurt
Juice of 1 lemon
Salt and pepper, to taste

## DIRECTIONS

1. In a blender, combine the peas, mint leaves, Greek yogurt, and lemon juice. Blend until smooth.
2. Season with salt and pepper to taste. Chill before serving as a refreshing dip.

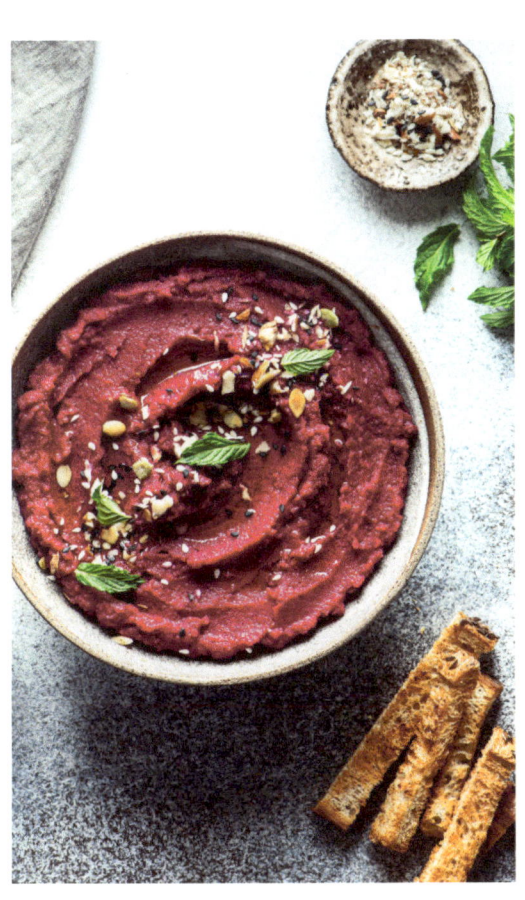

# CREAMY BEET HUMMUS

## INGREDIENTS

1 medium beet, roasted and peeled
1 can (15 oz) chickpeas, drained and rinsed
2 tablespoons tahini
2 cloves garlic
Juice of 1 lemon
2 tablespoons olive oil
Salt and pepper, to taste

## DIRECTIONS

1. Cut the roasted beet into chunks and add it to a blender along with the chickpeas, tahini, garlic, lemon juice, and olive oil.
2. Blend until smooth. Season with salt and pepper to taste.
3. Serve chilled as a vibrant, flavorful dip for soft bread or vegetables.

# CLASSIC GUACAMOLE

## INGREDIENTS

3 ripe avocados, mashed
Juice of 1 lime
1/2 teaspoon salt
1/2 teaspoon ground cumin (optional)
1/2 teaspoon crushed red pepper flakes (optional)
1/2 medium onion, finely diced
2 tomatoes, seeded and diced
1-2 cloves garlic, minced
2 tablespoons cilantro, chopped
1 jalapeño, seeded and minced (adjust to taste)

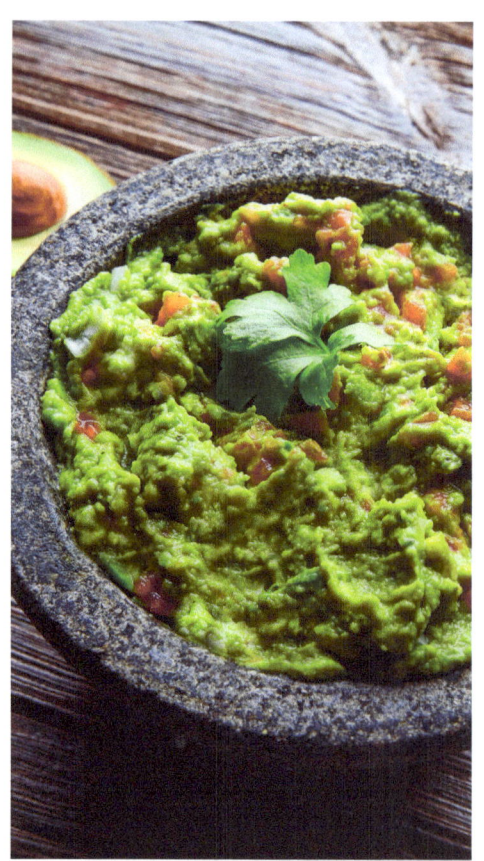

## DIRECTIONS

1. Cut the avocados in half and scoop the flesh into a mixing bowl. Use a fork to mash the avocado to a soft consistency
2. Squeeze the lime juice directly over the mashed avocado to prevent browning. Add the salt, cumin, red pepper, diced onion, minced garlic chopped cilantro, and minced jalapeño to the bowl. If you want a milder guacamole, you can reduce or omit the jalapeño.
3. Add diced tomatoes into the avocado mixture. This adds a fresh, slightly acidic taste that balances the creaminess of the avocado.
4. Stir well to combine all the flavors.

## A Table For Everyone

As you close this book, may you carry forward the spirit of creativity and adaptability in your kitchen. Whether you're cooking for a loved one with dietary restrictions or simply looking to expand your culinary repertoire, remember that food is a universal language of care and connection.

May your kitchen always be filled with laughter, love, and delectable aromas. Here's to many more meals that bring us together, no matter what challenges we may face.

Best wishes,
     Gabrielle Harper

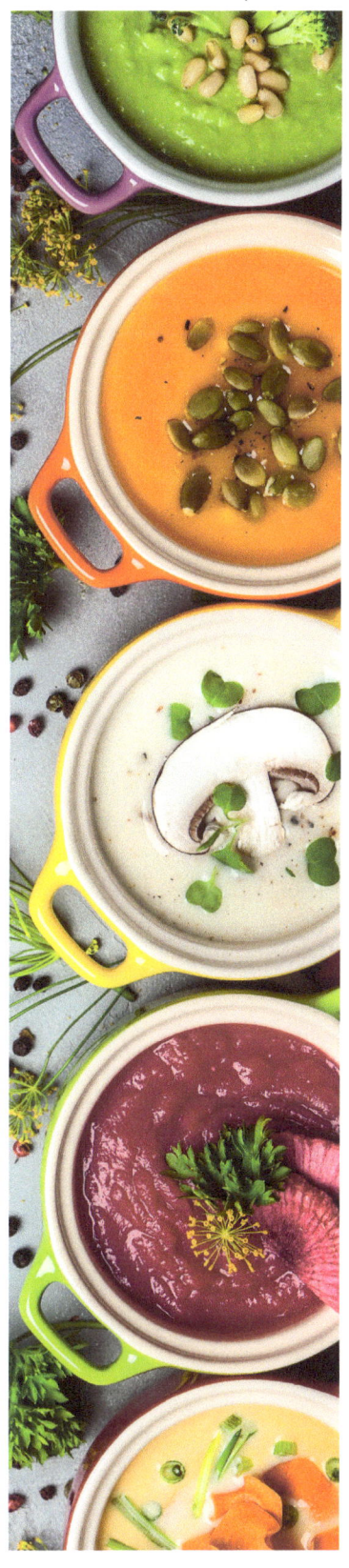

www.ingramcontent.com/pod-product-compliance
Lightning Source LLC
Chambersburg PA
CBHW040332220526
45473CB00009B/2660